# Table of Contents

# INTRODUCTION

Some weeks ago, the seers over at Google released a comprehensive report revealing the top trends in food and recipe search from coast to coast—offering, basically, a bird's eye view of Americans' culinary curiosities, guilty pleasures, and weeknight cravings. There were exciting up-and-comers on the list (turmeric, we're looking at you) and a few falling stars we won't miss (bacon cupcakes, anyone?) But the winner that put the biggest smile on our face was a classic Vietnamese dish that's a tricky to pronounce but super easy to slurp down: Pho.

Our affection for pho isn't entirely new: According to Google, searches for the fragrant noodle soup have increased steadily for the past decade, with a marked uptick—11 percent year-over-year—in the past three years alone. Certainly, if you've ever been to a Vietnamese restaurant, you've reveled in its heady aroma. While its origins are murky, most historians agree that pho first appeared around the turn of the 20th century in northern Vietnam, and some speculate that the name is a play on the French beef stew, pot au feu, which was introduced to the country during the period of colonization.

In its most basic form, a bowl of pho consists of a foundation of rice noodles topped with thinly sliced raw beef, which gets cooked when a portion of steaming, spiced beef broth is poured over top. Finished with a flurry of fresh herbs, like cilantro and basil, as well as crunchy bean sprouts, hot chiles, and tart lime, pho makes an, ahem, restorative meal any time of day. Indeed, in its home country, pho is still best loved as a breakfast dish, available from every corner food stall. But because, whether topped with beef or chicken, it is the robust, deeply savory broth that is its backbone, traditional versions of pho can take a day or more to make—there's just no faking that slow simmered stock. That's not exactly conducive to weeknight cooking, which is why most folks—even Vietnamese-Americans—usually buy their pho from a pro.

That may be changing, though. One of the more interesting details in Google's report explains that traffic around pho has recently included more recipe searches—suggesting that home cooks are eager to try and recreate the magic of the dish at home. We can certainly get behind that. And happily, as long as you're not a purist, there are plenty of pho shortcuts that deliver a lot of the deliciousness in a fraction of the time. Here, a few of our favorites:

Use store bought broth. Though there's no comparing the boxed stuff to the real thing, sometimes you just want a steaming bowl of pho right now. It pays to seek out a brand that is clean-tasting, rich, and beefy. Our fave? Trader Joe's Organic Beef Broth.

Add some exotic spices. Star anise, cloves, and cinnamon are the aromatic trinity in traditional pho stock—so try adding a few whole spices to the store-bought stuff, along with a bit of fresh ginger and a glug of funky fish sauce. Though it won't replicate the complexity of a long-simmered broth, it will infuse the mixture with a delightful aroma and deepen all of the flavors.

Use leftovers. Handling raw beef at the dinner table not your thing? Swap out the traditional topping for something a little more approachable (and convenient) like rotisserie chicken, leftover steak, or even Thanksgiving turkey. Vegetarian? Skip the meat and toss in some tofu or mushrooms instead.

Don't skimp on the add-ons. One of the best parts of traditional pho—the fresh garnishes—requires no cooking at all, so take the opportunity to really make them shine. Seek out the freshest, greenest basil and cilantro, a variety of chiles, the crunchiest sprouts, and the juiciest limes, and always offer plenty of them. Sriracha is also de rigeur—and hoisin sauce doesn't hurt either.

## CHAPTER ONE

**WHAT IS PHO AND WHAT IS IT MADE OF?**

Pho is a Vietnamese soup consisting of bone broth, rice noodles, and thinly sliced meat (usually beef). It may also be served with bean sprouts, fresh herbs, limes, chiles, and other garnishes. The origins of pho are a bit murky, but it is generally believed to have originated in early 20th century northern Vietnam. It eventually migrated south after the division of the country in 1954, and gained even more popularity following the Vietnam War as refugees introduced it to other cultures.

Traditionally, pho is prepared by simmering a broth made with beef bones, ginger, onions, and other spices over low heat for several hours. Rice noodles, known as "banh pho," are then added, as well as herbs like cilantro or basil. Finally, thinly sliced beef or chicken is incorporated and cooked in the hot broth. Some people like to top it with bean sprouts, vegetables, chili pepper, or lime. While most commonly eaten during the colder months, many restaurants serve this Vietnamese soup year round. Pho differs throughout Vietnam and in other parts of the world, depending on the broth's flavor, noodle size, and ingredients added to the finished product.

## HOW TO PRONOUNCE PHO

Here's a tidbit of information that will keep you from botching the pronunciation of this popular dish: Pho is pronounced "fuh" rather than "faux." You might find some subtle differences in pronunciation between the North and South Vietnamese, but "fuh" is the generally accepted pronunciation. The word "pho" actually comes from the French word "feu," meaning fire. This takes us back to the murky origin of pho — Vietnam was colonized by the French in the late 1880s, suggesting that pho could be a

Vietnamese rendition of the French dish pot au feu.

## TYPES OF PHO

When pho migrated south following the division of the country in 1954, it took on a new form. The result was two different types of pho, each belonging to a different region: pho bac and pho nam.

### PHO BAC

Considered the original pho, pho bac is northern Vietnamese pho. It's known for it's more mild, clear bone broth, wide noodles, and for the addition of lots of green onions.

### PHO NAM

Southern Vietnamese pho, called pho nam, is known for its bolder broth and thinner noodles. In the south, meat plays a larger role in pho, where it's common to use many parts of the cow including bone borrow, tendon, and brisket. It's typically topped with bean sprouts and fresh herbs.

This authentic pho recipe was adapted from Chef Eric of Ba Bar's pho recipe. Be sure to plan ahead — authentic pho requires six to 10 hours of cooking time for a flavorful bone broth. For best results, use shank and knee beef bones.

Ingredients:

- 4 pounds beef soup bones
- 1 onion, unpeeled and cut in half
- 5 slices fresh ginger
- 1 tablespoon salt
- 2 pods star anise
- 2 ½ tablespoons fish sauce
- 4 quarts water
- 1 (8 ounce) package dried rice noodles
- 1 ½ pounds beef top sirloin, thinly sliced
- ½ cup chopped cilantro
- 1 tablespoon chopped green onion
- 1 ½ cups bean sprouts
- 1 bunch Thai basil
- 1 lime, cut into 4 wedges
- ¼ cup hoisin sauce (Optional)

- ¼ cup chile-garlic sauce (such as Sriracha®) (Optional)

INSTRUCTIONS:

1. Preheat the oven to 425 degrees F (220 degrees C).
2. Place beef bones on a baking sheet and roast in the preheated oven until browned, about one hour.
3. Place onion on a baking sheet and roast in the preheated oven until blackened and soft, about 45 minutes.
4. Place bones, onion, ginger, salt, star anise, and fish sauce in a large stockpot and cover with four quarts of water. Bring to a boil and reduce heat to low. Simmer on low for six to 10 hours. Strain the broth into a saucepan and set aside.
5. Place rice noodles in a large bowl filled with room temperature water and allow to soak for one hour. Bring a large pot of water to a boil and after the noodles have soaked, place them in the boiling water for one minute. Bring stock to a simmer.

6. Divide noodles among four serving bowls; top with sirloin, cilantro, and green onion. Pour hot broth over the top. Stir and let sit until the beef is partially cooked and no longer pink, one to two minutes. Serve with bean sprouts, Thai basil, lime wedges, hoisin sauce, and chile-garlic sauce on the side.

## MORE WAYS TO MAKE PHO

While the above recipe is considered a traditional Vietnamese pho, we have loads of pho-inspired recipes like this easy My Chicken Pho recipe, or what's known as "pho ga," which is sometimes described as Vietnamese chicken noodle soup. For more recipe inspiration, browse our entire collection of Vietnamese Soups and Stews.

## PHO SOUP CAN BE FULL OF NUTRITION — AS LONG AS YOU'RE ORDERING OR MAKING IT THE RIGHT WAY

A blend of broth, rice noodles, herbs and meat (usually beef), pho soup is a common Vietnamese menu item. And like most restaurant foods, you need to be aware of how it's prepared and watch your portion sizes to make sure you're not overindulging. The amount of customization that can be done with a bowl of pho is part of what makes it so great. You can choose your protein (beef, chicken, tofu or tempeh), broth (vegetable, chicken or beef), veggies and noodles you want to add — there are a ton of different options.

This variety is also responsible for pho's nutrition.

BEEF PHO NUTRITION FACTS

A 20-ounce bowl of beef pho contains:

- Calories: 562
- Total fat: 4.7 g
- Cholesterol: 41 mg
- Sodium: 2,375 mg
- Total carbs: 104 g
- Dietary fiber: 6 g
- Sugar: 5 g
- Protein: 23 g

- Total fat: A 20-ounce bowl of beef pho has 4.7 grams of total fat, which includes 3.2 grams of unsaturated fat, 1.5 grams of saturated fat and 0 grams of trans fat.
- Carbohydrates: A 20-ounce bowl of beef pho has 104 grams of carbs, which includes 6 grams of fiber and 5 grams of sugar.
- Protein: A 20-ounce bowl of beef pho has 23 grams of protein.

## VITAMINS, MINERALS AND OTHER MICRONUTRIENTS

- Vitamin C: 44% Daily Value (DV)
- Vitamin A: 24% DV
- Iron: 17% DV
- Calcium: 8%

## HEALTH BENEFITS OF BEEF PHO

Pho supplies several key vitamins and minerals and is an ample source of protein. Pho soup can certainly fit into a healthy eating plan, especially if you prepare it at home, and include some of the healthier protein, broth, noodle and vegetable options.

Protein is an essential macronutrient, which helps grow and maintain our muscles, tendons, blood vessels, hair, nails and skin, according to the Academy of Nutrition and Dietetics. The macronutrient is also vital for creating enzymes and hormones, all of which help our bodies function properly. A serving of beef pho provides 24 grams of protein. The Institute of Medicine recommends keeping your protein intake to 10 to 35 percent of your total caloric intake, and pho can help you reach that goal.

## IT'S AN EXCELLENT SOURCE OF VITAMINS A AND C

Pho can be packed with vitamins. A 20-ounce bowl of beef pho provides 24 percent of your recommended daily allowance of vitamin A and 44 percent of vitamin C. Vitamin A is a fat soluble vitamin that is important for normal vision and helping your heart, kidneys and lungs function properly, according to the National Institutes of Health (NIH). The vitamin is also an antioxidant that works to protect your body from free radicals like pollution, smoke and UV lights from the sun. Vitamin A supports your immune and reproductive systems as well. Vitamin C is a water soluble vitamin and antioxidant — it also helps to protect your body from free radicals, according to the NIH. Vitamin C also supports our immune system, aids in wound healing and increases the absorption of iron in our bodies.

### BEEF PHO IS A GREAT SOURCE OF IRON

One of the most notable nutrients in pho soup is iron, although this can vary depending on the protein source and added vegetables and broth. A serving of beef pho contains 17 percent of the daily value for iron. Iron is a mineral that our bodies rely on for proper growth and development, according to the NIH. Our bodies need iron to make hemoglobin, a protein found in red blood cells, which transports oxygen throughout our body. This is why people who are iron-deficient typically feel fatigued. Pho may just seem like a basic soup, but its ingredients may offer various benefits.

Many of the ingredients in pho offer potential health benefits, such as:

- Bone broth may promote joint health. Bone broth contains glucosamine, chondroitin, and collagen — all of which may promote joint health. Yet, it typically provides only small amounts of these substances.
- Ginger helps reduce inflammation. Ginger contains gingerol, a compound that has been shown to have anti-inflammatory and antioxidant effects and may reduce joint pain and inflammation.
- Herbs and vegetables are highly nutritious. Herbs and vegetables in pho, such as Thai basil, cilantro, green onions, and chili peppers, pack many nutrients and potent anti-inflammatory compounds.

## GOOD SOURCE OF PROTEIN

Most variations of pho include either beef, pork, chicken, or tofu. A 2-cup (475ml) serving packs about 30 grams of protein, making it an excellent source of this filling nutrient. Sufficient protein intake is important, as this macronutrient serves as the main building block for your body and is used to make muscles, tendons, organs, skin, and hormones. It's also needed for other processes. The recommended dietary allowance for protein is 0.4 grams per pound (0.8 grams per kg) of body weight per day, though most people require more than that. Eating pho as part of a healthy diet can help you meet your needs.

*CONTAINS NUTRIENT-RICH HERBS*

Many spices and herbs, including cilantro and basil in pho, are high in polyphenols. These compounds have been linked to a reduced risk of chronic conditions like heart disease and cancer. Though it's difficult to determine the amount of herbs and spices needed to reap health benefits, eating pho can contribute to your intake of these powerful substances.

*GLUTEN-FREE*

As rice noodles are typically used in pho, the dish is often gluten-free — though this also depends on other ingredients and how they were processed. While a gluten-free diet is not necessarily healthier, pho can be a good option if you avoid gluten. The nutrient-dense ingredients in pho may reduce inflammation and chronic disease risk. Plus, the dish is generally gluten-free.

## POTENTIAL DOWNSIDES

Though eating pho may offer certain benefits, you should look out for a few things.

### CAN BE HIGH IN SODIUM

Pho can be high in sodium, especially commercially prepared versions. Soup bases and broths tend to be high in sodium, providing close to 1,000 mg per 1-cup (240-ml) serving. The Dietary Guidelines for Americans, published by the Department of Health and Human Services and Department of Agriculture, recommend no more than 2,300 mg daily. Thus, just one serving of pho could pack about half of your daily sodium allowance. Consuming too much sodium can have negative health effects in certain populations, the most notable being increased blood pressure. The best way to reduce the sodium content of pho is to make the bone broth from scratch or buy a lower-sodium variety.



The calorie content of pho can vary greatly depending on the type of noodles and cut of meat used. To keep calories in check, use a rice noodle that's higher in fiber, such as those made with brown rice. Added fiber can help promote feelings of fullness, making you eat fewer calories overall. Fiber and nutrient contents can also be increased by including more vegetables, such as mushrooms, carrots, bean sprouts, or dark leafy greens. To control added fat and calories from meat, use a leaner cut of beef, such as top round. Leaner protein options, such as chicken or tofu, work well, too.

Incorporating more vegetables and lean protein and reducing the amount of noodles in your pho can help fill you up more quickly, which may reduce overeating. Pho can be high in sodium and calories depending on the ingredients used. Make bone broth from scratch or use a low-sodium variety, and focus on leaner protein sources and high-fiber noodles.

## BEEF PHO HEALTH RISKS

While pho has some healthy attributes, it has some downsides as well.

### SODIUM

Sodium content can vary greatly, again, depending on the type of protein and broth used. A serving of beef pho has 2,375 milligrams, or about 100 percent of the Daily Value. A high-sodium diet can raise your blood pressure, which leaves you at a greater risk for heart attack and stroke, according to the American Heart Association. If you are concerned about your sodium intake as many are with high blood pressure, there are ways to make pho lower in sodium.NA few options would be to make your own broth (you can do so with water as a base and add salt to your own liking), use meat or proteins that are not salted, use a salt-free seasoning and/or limit the use of additional sauces like hoisin and sriracha.

A 20-ounce bowl of beef pho has 104 grams of carbohydrates. This equates to about seven slices of bread. Rice noodles are a refined carbohydrate so there's minimal fiber and nutrients. Case in point: This 20-ounce serving has just 6 grams of fiber.

Our bodies need carbohydrates but you want to choose your carbs wisely. In place of refined carbs like white rice noodles, which have been stripped of the majority of their fiber and other nutrients, opt for whole-grain pasta instead. And stick to one serving of pasta per bowl.

## FOOD ALLERGIES

The top nine food allergies are milk, egg, peanut, soy, wheat, shellfish, fish, sesame and tree nuts. Adding an egg is common when ordering pho so if you have an egg allergy, you'll want to refrain from having it added.

Additionally, fish sauce, sesame oil and peanuts/peanut oil are popular at Vietnamese restaurants so you'll want to ensure they're not used in the cooking, as a garnish, or that your dish hasn't been prepared near these foods if you have an allergy.


DRUG INTERACTIONS

The potential food and drug interactions depend on what you decide to include in your pho. If you add a high amount of leafy greens, more than you're used to consuming, they could interact with blood thinning medications like warfarin or coumadin. To be safe, ask health care provider if the medications you're on interact with any foods or beverages.

HOW TO ORDER OR MAKE HEALTHIER PHO

While the occasional serving of pho soup at a restaurant can have a place in your diet, there are modifications you can make to your order to make it healthier, or try making your own at home. Here are a few tips:

- Load up on the veggies. "When making pho at home, I recommend adding plenty of vegetables as this will not only enhance the flavor but will also increase the nutrient content of your pho," Ligos shares. When ordering pho away from home, Ligos recommends asking for a variety of vegetable and topping options (like bean sprouts) to make sure you're getting plenty of nutritious vitamins and minerals.

- Switch up the noodles. The best noodles for pho are made of rice, but swapping those rice noodles for noodles higher in fiber, such as whole-wheat, is another way to boost the nutrition of the soup.

- Cut down on salt. "Be careful what broth you use. I recommend either making your own or searching for a low-sodium brand to ensure you can control how much sodium goes into the pho," Ligos says.

- Add all the herbs. Fresh herbs, such as cilantro or basil, deliver a small boost of vitamin A, and a squirt of fresh lime juice adds a bit of vitamin C. Skip the salty hot sauces in favor of fresh jalapeno, which is naturally sodium-free.

- Go for leaner sources of protein. "I also recommend adding some sort of protein whether chicken, beef or tofu to ensure the dish is filling and fully satisfying. You might even consider adding a soft-boiled egg at the end," Ligos shares.

## IS PHO HEALTHY OR NOT? WILL I GAIN WEIGHT IF I HAVE IT OFTEN?

A warm bowl of pho soup is everyone's favorite these days. Made with a blend of broth, meat, rice noodles, and topped with vegetables, pho has it all from a nutritional standpoint. But there's also talk about pho being unhealthy due to its high sodium content and that it was even fattening. Whether pho is good or bad for you depends on the specific recipe, your choice of condiments, and portion size.

Many of us tend to go overboard with our portion sizes when given a variety of options of meat, veggies etc.

Most of us have had their first bowl pho at our local Vietnamese restaurants where customers are given a variety of options of meat, veggies, serving size, and condiments. No wonder, so many of us tend to go overboard with our portion sizes with that much freedom available. You've probably asked yourself at one point is pho healthy and will it ruin your waistline? This is especially true if you eat pho on an almost daily basis and feel guilty about it. Another thing that may make you feel weary about pho is that you don't see this traditionally Vietnamese dish being recommended as a weight-loss and health promoting option. Instead, you are more likely to hear pho referred to as an unhealthy fast-food or street-food.

Hearing talk of pho being one of those unhealthy restaurant meals can kill all the fun around this popular noodle soup. Well, we're here to tell you that pho can be a big part of even the best diet plan if you eat it moderately and if you customize it wisely. On the downside, many low-quality restaurant versions tend to be high in saturated fat and sodium, so this can get a bit tricky. Studies show that too much fat in your diet can lead to weight gain, a higher risk of diabetes, and cardiovascular disease. Furthermore, too much sodium in your daily diet can cause hypertension and damage your heart, kidneys, and blood vessels.



Americans have been slurping down pho, a hearty Vietnamese noodle soup, increasingly for the past decade, but a big question remains: Is pho healthy?

There's nothing quite like a big, steaming bowl of pho (pronounced "fuh")—typically made up of a meaty broth, white rice flour noodles, beef or chicken, and spices and topped with a medley of herbs, bean sprouts, hot chiles, and a lime— on an icy winter day or night. (In Vietnam, it's usually eaten for breakfast like Cheerios.) It's deeply comforting and filling, but you don't walk away from the meal feeling stuffed as you might after eating a meal of pizza and pasta or fried foods. But if you have ever wondered if it's good for you, or even detoxifying like other types of bone broth soups, you are definitely not alone. We consulted the experts to weigh in.

Pho is a very nutritious dish. Made with rice noodles and a rich beef bone stock, it's a perfect vehicle for bean sprouts and nutrient-rich herbs. The soup itself, a rich bone broth, is filled with health benefits for your body, including your immune and digestive system, and your bones and joints. In terms of calorie content, pho ranges from 350 to about 500 calories on average depending on the size of the portion and the meat or even seafood you add in. Pho is a great source of protein (vital for your bones, muscles, cartilage, skin and blood), When it comes to the protein, opt for lean cuts of meat or veggies to lower your saturated fat intake. Eating foods that contain high levels of saturated fat regularly can raise blood cholesterol which increases your risk of heart disease. Chicken is leaner than beef.

The noodle soup has also been cited by doctors as an excellent cold remedy due to all the healing spices it's packed with, such as coriander and anise. Rice noodles don't offer much in the way of nutritional value, so swapping them out for brown rice noodles to make your pho healthier. While it may not be traditional, at home, you can get more nutrition out of your pho by using brown rice noodles for more fiber.

Adding veggies, such as carrots, broccoli or spinach, to your pho is another great way to increase the nutrition in your bowl. "Fresh vegetables added to pho are a nutritious addition," says Syn. "Vegetables are low in calories and high in vitamins, minerals and filling fiber. The one thing to be extra conscientious with pho is that it's very high in sodium, which can cause increased blood pressure and contribute to cardiovascular issues. (Some bowls have more than 1,000 mg, which is practically the entire allotment of recommended sodium intake for the day.) "Depending on the broth used and amount of fish sauce added, sodium can add up quickly. Making pho at home with a low-sodium stock as a good alternative or pairing it with a lower sodium side, like a salad of fresh cucumbers dressed in rice vinegar and sesame oil with herbs.

While pho may come with its downsides, you can customize this delicious Vietnamese dish to make it more healthful. Compared to other fast-food dishes, a small serving of pho is quite balanced in nutrients and pretty low in calories. For instance, an appetizer serving size of chicken pho contains only 162 calories. Of this, 32% of the calories come from fat, 32% come from carbohydrates, and 36% of the calories in one cup of pho come from protein. On the other hand, a meal-sized portion of pho may provide up to 400 calories which are only 20% of the recommended daily intake of calories.

As you can see, good quality pho isn't the highly fattening fast food it was made up to be. This is especially true with pho that was made using traditional methods. Traditionally, pho was made by cooking beef bones or chicken for a very long time, and the excess fat at the top was removed. Restaurant versions may skip this last step, but high-end restaurants make it a priority to make their meals healthy and delicious. But other than providing you with a modest number of calories, pho is also great for meeting your vitamin and mineral needs. Pho is rich in vitamin A, vitamin C, calcium, and iron. Depending on how much veggies you like to include, you can also get plenty of fiber from your bowl of pho.



Enjoying pho and getting plenty of health benefits with it is possible is you make the right decisions. First, it is best to look for a Vietnamese restaurant serving traditional pho instead of the fast-food version. As we've already explained, some restaurants skip skimming the excess fat from their pho broth making for an unhealthier soup version. Secondly, when customizing your pho at your favorite restaurant, be careful no tot go overboard with certain ingredients. Too much rice noodles will cause a spike in your blood glucose and make a meal fattening. Similarly, adding more than your fair share of meat cuts to your bowl of pho will pack on the extra calories. Instead, be generous with vegetable topping when customizing your pho. Veggies like bean sprouts, jalapenos, and onions will control your blood glucose levels, and their fiber content will keep you feeling full.

But other than customizing your pho bowl to suit your health-conscious lifestyle, why not play it safe and make a homemade version instead? While Pho is traditionally made over the course of one to two days, there are plenty pho recipes requiring just a fraction of that time. With homemade pho, you get to have more control over the amount of fat, protein, and carbs you consume with each portion. We suggest opting for homemade chicken pho because chicken is leaner than beef.

We also suggest being moderate with condiments like soy sauce and siracha sauce. While these sauces help make pho taste great, they are very high in sodium. Restaurant versions also tend to go overboard with the sodium in pho to make it more palatable. But as already explained, this practice can be dangerous for your overall health. Instead, add only a tiny bit of sauces and salt to your pho, just enough to remove any blandness. You can also be playful with your topping and add spring onions or broccoli even. Make sure to read about low-calorie foods and benefits of broccoli before making your homemade pho.

Whether or not pho is healthy varies greatly from one version to the other. Traditional pho served with skimmed broth, a moderate serving of noodles, a tiny bit of sauce, and a generous helping of veggies is nutritious and possibly healthy. On the other hand, fast-food versions packed in sodium and saturated fat may not be the best choice for a daily meal. To get around this problem, pho lovers can customize their bowls by adding more veggies, being skimpy with condiments, and adding noodles moderately.

## PHO VS RAMEN: THE DIFFERENCE BETWEEN THESE SOUPS

One can draw quite a distinction between pho vs ramen, but it's come to the attention that not everyone does. When I was looking for a place to eat with my dad last week, I pointed out a pho place across the street and asked if he'd ever had pho. He said he had and reminded me of the restaurant Urban Ramen that we went to in California (which literally has ramen in the name). He asked what the difference was between pho vs ramen and I couldn't really explain it, so I looked into the facts.

Just so nobody else ever has to get stuck in the debate of pho vs ramen, I'm about to break down each dish and show you what makes them each unique. If you've tasted both, you know that they really aren't the same at all. If you haven't, I understand your confusion.


Pho (pronounced "fuh") is a Vietnamese soup made with broth, rice noodles, and usually some form of sliced meat. I prefer my pho simple with only chicken, but most people go with beef. A bowl of pho usually comes with a side of fresh herbs, lime and crunchy bean sprouts to top off your soup.

The origin of pho is a bit iffy. Some people believe it was derived from Mongolian Hot Pot, while others think the Vietnamese brought it over from China's Yunnan Province, where they went to flee French occupation. Regardless of how it got to Vietnam, we know that this soup is a staple of Vietnamese cooking and a popular street food.


## WHAT IS RAMEN?

Ramen, on the other hand, is a popular Japanese dish. It was originally imported from China but has become a staple in Japanese cuisine. Ramen dishes can be made from many different types of broth including Miso, Shoyu (Soy Sauce), Shio (Salt), and Tonkotsu (Pork Bone.) Although ramen can come with a variety of noodles, the most common are those curly ones we all know and love. Yes, like the ones you get from an instant noodle package. Or like JT's 90's 'do

I think the most noticeable difference between pho vs ramen is the toppings. Whereas pho is usually more minimalistic with herbs and sprouts, ramen has a long list of ingredients that normally go with the soup. Common toppings include roasted pork, a hard or soft boiled egg, seaweed, sprouts, corn, and narutomaki (the little white disk with the pink swirl).


Besides the origins, the difference between pho vs ramen is mostly in the noodle and the topping. Both start with a broth (although ramen has more common variations of broth), but you can instantly tell the difference by looking at those noodles. Pho noodles are rice noodles, so they're translucent and light. Ramen noodles, however, have a special ingredient: kansui. Kansui is a form of alkaline water originally from Mongolia, which is said to give ramen noodles that firm texture.

The other big difference is the toppings. Although they can both vary tremendously in toppings, there are some staples that make each of them unique. The meat in pho is sliced quite thinly, whereas the meat in ramen is usually thicker and fattier. The egg is also a key part of a bowl of ramen, something you really wouldn't find in the Vietnamese soup. Personally, I find ramen to be packed with more flavor and the broth tends to be a bit thicker than pho.

I know I said there are a lot of ramen options, but if you've ever been to a pho restaurant you know the menu can be endless. I'm sure there are some variations of both soups that are similar to each other, but when we get down to the root of the dish, the two soups are very different and have very different flavor profiles.

Now that you know the difference, go out and try both for yourself. Both are warm, cozy, and the perfect lunch to get you through a cold winter day. Both soups are also usually pretty cheap, so a pho or ramen date is a great way to hang out with friends on a budget. These soups are also great for late night/drunk eats. You may not find yourself craving soup after a night out, but once you try it you'll be craving it all the time.

## CHAPTER TWO

## Authentic Pho

This authentic pho isn't quick, but it is delicious. The key is in the broth, which gets simmered for at least 6 hours.

Prep: 20 mins

Cook: 8 hrs

Additional: 1 hr

Total: 9 hrs 20 mins

Servings: 4

Yield: 4 servings

Ingredients

4 pounds beef soup bones

1 onion, unpeeled and cut in half

5 slices fresh ginger

1 tablespoon salt

2 pods star anise

2 ½ tablespoons fish sauce

4 quarts water

1 (8 ounce) package dried rice noodles

1 ½ pounds beef top sirloin, thinly sliced

½ cup chopped cilantro

1 tablespoon chopped green onion

1 ½ cups bean sprouts

1 bunch Thai basil

1 lime, cut into 4 wedges

¼ cup hoisin sauce (Optional)

¼ cup chile-garlic sauce (such as Sriracha®) (Optional)

Directions

Step 1

Preheat oven to 425 degrees F (220 degrees C).

Step 2

Place beef bones on a baking sheet and roast in the preheated oven until browned, about 1 hour.

Step 3

Place onion on a baking sheet and roast in the preheated oven until blackened and soft, about 45 minutes.

Step 4

Place bones, onion, ginger, salt, star anise, and fish sauce in a large stockpot and cover with 4 quarts of water. Bring to a boil and reduce heat to low. Simmer on low for 6 to 10 hours. Strain the broth into a saucepan and set aside.

Step 5

Place rice noodles in large bowl filled with room temperature water and allow to soak for 1 hour. Bring a large pot of water to a boil and after the noodles have soaked, place them in the boiling water for 1 minute. Bring stock to a simmer.

Step 6

Divide noodles among 4 serving bowls; top with sirloin, cilantro, and green onion. Pour hot broth over the top. Stir and let sit until the beef is partially cooked and no longer pink, 1 to 2 minutes. Serve with bean sprouts, Thai basil, lime wedges, hoisin sauce, and chile-garlic sauce on the side.

Nutrition Facts

Per Serving: 209 calories; protein 34.9g; carbohydrates 65.6g; fat 11g; cholesterol 74mg; sodium 3519.3mg.

## Authentic Oxtail Pho

This oxtail pho recipe is authentic. This is the way my husband's family has always made it and it is delicious. My kids have grown up on this comforting noodle soup, which is especially good on a cold rainy day. Garnish with hoisin sauce and sriracha as desired.

Prep: 20 mins

Cook: 6 hrs 5 mins

Total: 6 hrs 25 mins

Servings: 8

Yield: 8 servings

Ingredients

water to cover

1 ½ pounds beef oxtail, or to taste

2 Spanish onions, peeled, divided

1 tablespoon fish sauce, or to taste

1 tablespoon whole star anise pods

1 cinnamon stick

salt to taste

3 tablespoons beef pho flavor paste

2 bunches scallions, chopped

1 bunch fresh cilantro, chopped

1 (16 ounce) package dried rice noodles, or to taste

1 (12 ounce) package beef pho meatballs, halved, or to taste

½ pound sirloin steak, thinly sliced, or to taste

1 lime, cut into 8 wedges

4 teaspoons white sugar, or to taste

1 (8 ounce) package bean sprouts

1 bunch Thai basil leaves, torn into bite-size pieces

1 (2.8 ounce) can crispy fried shallots, or to taste

Directions

Step 1

Bring water and oxtail to a boil in a pot. Skim the foam and oil off the surface. Add 1 onion, fish sauce, star anise, cinnamon, and salt. Stir in pho flavor paste; cover loosely with a lid. Reduce heat and simmer broth for at least 6 hours.

Step 2

Cut the remaining onion in half and slice very thinly. Place in a bowl with scallions and cilantro.

Step 3

Place noodles in a large bowl and rinse. Cover with warm water and let soak for 1 hour.

Step 4

Drop meatballs into the soup 20 minutes before broth is done.

Step 5

Bring a small saucepan of water to a boil. Drain noodles and dip into the boiling water for 30 seconds. Transfer noodles into 8 large bowls.

Step 6

Top each bowl with sliced sirloin. Ladle in broth, meatballs, and oxtail. Taste and season as needed. Squeeze 1 or 2 lime wedges into each bowl and mix in 1/2 teaspoon sugar. Top with the cilantro-onion mixture, bean sprouts, basil, and shallots.

Nutrition Facts

Per Serving: 267 calories; protein 30.4g; carbohydrates 69.7g; fat 18.3g; cholesterol 91.8mg; sodium 743.8mg.

### Chicken Pho

Mom's chicken pho recipe... straight from Vietnam. Serve with hoisin and sriracha sauce.

Prep: 30 mins

Cook: 1 hr 30 mins

Total: 2 hrs

Servings: 24

Yield: 24 servings

Ingredients

10 quarts water

3 pounds chicken bones

1 whole chicken

1 medium onion

1 (1 inch) piece ginger

1 (32 fluid ounce) container chicken broth

¼ cup rock sugar

3 teaspoons fish sauce

2 cubes pho ga soup seasoning

1 ½ teaspoons salt

2 (16 ounce) packages rice stick noodles (banh pho)

½ pound bean sprouts

1 bunch green onion, chopped

1 bunch cilantro, chopped

6 sprigs Thai basil, or as needed

1 lime, cut in wedges

Directions

Step 1

Bring water to a boil in a stockpot. Meanwhile, rinse chicken bones under hot water to get rid of impurities.

Step 2

Place bones in the pot of boiling water. Reduce heat and simmer until starting to soften, skimming any fat off the surface of the broth, about 60 minutes. Discard parboiled bones.

Step 3

Place whole chicken into the pot and simmer until no longer pink in the center, 30 to 40 minutes. Remove chicken from broth and set aside to cool. An instant-read thermometer inserted near the bone should read 165 degrees F (74 degrees C).

Step 4

Combine onion and ginger in a skillet over medium-high heat. Cook and stir until nicely browned and fragrant, about 7 minutes. Smash ginger with the backside of a knife onto a cutting board. Place onion and ginger into the broth.

Add chicken broth, rock sugar, fish sauce, pho ga seasoning, and salt.

Step 5

Bring a large pot of water to a boil. Add rice noodles and boil until tender yet firm to the bite, 2 to 3 minutes. Drain.

Step 6

Peel skin off of the cooled chicken; discard skin and bones, reserving the meat.

Step 7

Serve noodles in bowls topped with chicken meat and broth. Garnish with bean sprouts, green onion, cilantro, and Thai basil. Squeeze a wedge of lime into each bowl.

Nutrition Facts

Per Serving: 224 calories; protein 19.9g; carbohydrates 34.1g; fat 11.1g; cholesterol 72.5mg; sodium 520mg.

## Amanda's Quick Pho

Based off of recipe for Vietnamese pho, with a twist. Easy enough to make at home and good enough to forego takeout. Garnish with generous helpings of cilantro, bean sprouts, fresh basil, additional hoisin sauce, and sriracha hot sauce.

Prep: 10 mins

Cook: 10 mins

Additional: 15 mins

Total: 35 mins

Servings: 10

Yield: 3 quarts

Ingredients

3 quarts fat-free chicken broth

1 onion, sliced into rings

2 tablespoons hoisin sauce

1 tablespoon oyster sauce

1 tablespoon minced garlic

½ teaspoon ginger powder

½ teaspoon curry powder

1 pinch ground cinnamon

1 (16 ounce) package dried rice noodles

1 roasted chicken

Directions

Step 1

Combine broth, onion, hoisin sauce, oyster sauce, garlic, ginger, curry, and cinnamon in a saucepan. Bring to a boil, reduce heat, and simmer until onions are tender, about 5 minutes.

Step 2

Place noodles in a large bowl and cover with hot water. Set aside until noodles are softened, about 15 minutes. Drain and rinse thoroughly.

Step 3

Pull meat from roasted chicken and thickly shred. Add to broth. Spoon broth and chicken over noodles.

Nutrition Facts

Per Serving: 283 calories; protein 20.4g; carbohydrates 40.2g; fat 3.4g; cholesterol 34.1mg; sodium 646.9mg.

## Pho

This is a shortened and easier version of the delicious Vietnamese soup called Pho Bac. Garnish with pepper, green chiles, hoisin sauce, chili sauce and lime wedges.

Prep: 30 mins

Cook: 4 hrs 30 mins

Total: 5 hrs

Servings: 3

Yield: 3 servings

Ingredients

4 pounds bone-in beef shank

1 onion

5 slices fresh ginger root

1 pod star anise, whole

1 teaspoon salt

2 ½ tablespoons fish sauce

1 (8 ounce) package dried rice noodles

½ pound cooked beef sirloin, thinly sliced

3 green onions, chopped

1 ½ cups fresh bean sprouts

6 sprigs cilantro

Directions

Step 1

In a large pot over medium heat, bring beef shank and 3 quarts water to a boil. Skim off foam. Reduce heat, cover and simmer 4 hours.

Step 2

Preheat oven broiler. Place unpeeled whole onion under broiler until soft. Remove and peel.

Step 3

Stir onion, ginger, anise, salt and fish sauce into beef mixture.

Step 4

Bring a large pot of lightly salted water to a boil. Add rice noodles and cook for 8 to 10 minutes or until al dente; drain.

Step 5

Divide noodles into three serving bowls. Place cooked sirloin on top of pasta in bowls. Sprinkle green onions, bean sprouts and cilantro evenly in bowls. Strain beef broth and divide evenly between serving bowls, pouring over assembled ingredients. Serve at once.

Nutrition Facts

Per Serving: 210 calories; protein 107.7g; carbohydrates 54.7g; fat 46.8g; cholesterol 267mg; sodium 1938.5mg.

**Vietnamese Beef Pho**

This soup is served with a plate full of fresh garnishes as well as various sauces. This allows each person to season their serving to taste. The soup is somewhat unusual, because the meat is cooked in the bowl. The beef is sliced very thin, almost thin enough to see through. You might want to have the butcher slice it for you. The boiling hot broth is poured over the noodles and raw meat. The meat is quickly cooked in the hot broth in the time it takes to garnish the soup.

Prep: 10 mins

Cook: 1 hr 20 mins

Total: 1 hr 30 mins

Servings: 6

Yield: 6 servings

Ingredients

4 quarts beef broth

1 large onion, sliced into rings

6 slices fresh ginger root

1 lemon grass

1 cinnamon stick

1 teaspoon whole black peppercorns

1 pound sirloin tip, cut into thin slices

½ pound bean sprouts

1 cup fresh basil leaves

1 cup fresh mint leaves

1 cup loosely packed cilantro leaves

3 fresh jalapeno peppers, sliced into rings

2 limes, cut into wedges

2 (8 ounce) packages dried rice noodles

½ tablespoon hoisin sauce

1 dash hot pepper sauce

3 tablespoons fish sauce

Directions

Step 1

In a large soup pot, combine broth, onion, ginger, lemon grass, cinnamon, and peppercorns. Bring to a boil, reduce heat, and cover. Simmer for 1 hour.

Step 2

Arrange bean sprouts, mint, basil, and cilantro on a platter with chilies and lime.

Step 3

Soak the noodles in hot water to cover for 15 minutes or until soft. Drain. Place equal portions of noodles into 6 large soup bowls, and place raw beef on top. Ladle hot broth over noodles and beef. Pass platter with garnishes and sauces.

Nutrition Facts

Per Serving: 228 calories; protein 27.1g; carbohydrates 73.1g; fat 13.6g; cholesterol 50.7mg; sodium 2843.8mg.

## Chicken Zoodle Pho

Chicken zoodle pho made super simple in the slow cooker and topped with spiralized zucchini noodles for a healthy version of a restaurant favorite. Make takeout easy at home with a comforting bowl of this gluten-free and low-calorie soup!

Prep: 20 mins

Cook: 2 hrs 30 mins

Total: 2 hrs 50 mins

Servings: 6

Yield: 6 servings

Ingredients

10 cups vegetable broth

12 ounces boneless chicken breasts

1 ½ cups sliced white onion, separated into rings

2 tablespoons oyster sauce

1 ½ teaspoons coconut sugar

1 teaspoon salt

1 teaspoon ground black pepper

4 whole cloves

½ teaspoon minced ginger

2 whole star anise pods

9 cups bean sprouts

6 cups coarsely chopped bok choy cabbage

4 zucchini

Directions

Step 1

Combine vegetable broth, chicken breasts, onions, oyster sauce, coconut sugar, salt, pepper, cloves, ginger, and star anise in a slow cooker.

Step 2

Cook on High until chicken breasts can be easily flaked with a fork, about 1 1/2 hour. Stir in bean sprouts and bok choy. Continue cooking soup until bean sprouts are tender, about 1 hour.

Step 3

Cut zucchini into thin noodles using a spiralizer.

Step 4

Divide soup among 6 serving bowls. Top with zucchini noodles.

Nutrition Facts

Per Serving: 180 calories; protein 18.2g; carbohydrates 23.3g; fat 2.6g; cholesterol 29.3mg; sodium 1277.5mg.

## Beef Pho

Authentic South Vietnamese Style Pho. A comforting richly seasoned beef broth is ladled over rice noodles and thinly sliced beef. Add hot sauce and plum sauce to taste and top with cilantro, basil, lime juice and bean sprouts.

Prep: 30 mins

Cook: 6 hrs

Total: 6 hrs 30 mins

Servings: 6

Yield: 6 servings

Ingredients

5 pounds beef knuckle, with meat

2 pounds beef oxtail

1 white (daikon) radish, sliced

2 onions, chopped

2 ounces whole star anise pods

½ cinnamon stick

2 whole cloves

1 teaspoon black peppercorns

1 slice fresh ginger root

1 tablespoon white sugar

1 tablespoon salt

1 tablespoon fish sauce

1 ½ pounds dried flat rice noodles

½ pound frozen beef sirloin

TOPPINGS:

Sriracha hot pepper sauce

hoisin sauce

thinly sliced onion

chopped fresh cilantro

bean sprouts (mung beans)

sweet Thai basil

thinly sliced green onion

limes, quartered

Directions

Step 1

Place the beef knuckle in a very large (9 quart or more) pot. Season with salt, and fill pot with 2 gallons of water. Bring to a boil, and cook for about 2 hours.

Step 2

Skim fat from the surface of the soup, and add the oxtail, radish and onions. Tie the anise pods, cinnamon stick, cloves, peppercorns and ginger in a cheesecloth or place in a spice bag; add to the soup. Stir in sugar, salt and fish sauce. Simmer over medium-low heat for at least 4 more hours (the longer, the better). At the end of cooking, taste, and add salt as needed. Strain broth, and return to the pot to keep at a simmer. Discard spices and bones. Reserve meat from the beef knuckle for other uses if desired.

Step 3

Bring a large pot of lightly salted water to a boil. Soak the rice noodles in water for about 20 minutes, then cook in boiling water until soft, but not mushy, about 5 minutes. Slice the frozen beef paper thin. The meat must be thin enough to cook instantly.

Step 4

Place some noodles into each bowl, and top with a few raw beef slices. Ladle boiling broth over the beef and noodles in the bowl. Serve with hoisin sauce and Sriracha sauce on the side. Set onion, cilantro, bean sprouts, basil, green onions, and lime out at the table for individuals to add toppings to their liking.

Nutrition Facts

Per Serving: 214 calories; protein 139.3g; carbohydrates 101.6g; fat 35.7g; cholesterol 484.6mg; sodium 2101.2mg.

### Phoritto (Pho + Burrito)

All your favorite flavors of pho... in a tortilla! I get the meat, broth, noodles, and Thai basil from my local Asian grocery market.

Prep: 25 mins

Cook: 20 mins

Total: 45 mins

Servings: 8

Yield: 8 phorittos

Ingredients

1 tablespoon vegetable oil

1 ½ onion, thinly sliced

3 jalapeno peppers, thinly sliced

2 (14 ounce) cans beef-flavored pho broth

1 pound frozen ribeye steak, thinly sliced

10 ounces thin rice noodles (vermicelli-style)

8 burrito-size flour tortillas

1 (8 ounce) jar chili-garlic sauce

1 (8 ounce) package bean sprouts

2 tablespoons hoisin sauce, or to taste

1 bunch Thai basil

1 bunch cilantro

1 lime, sliced

Directions

Step 1

Heat oil in a large saucepan over medium heat. Add onions; cook and stir until softened, about 5 minutes. Add jalapenos; cook and stir until dark green, about 5 minutes. Remove from heat.

Step 2

Heat broth in a saucepan over medium-high heat. Cook batches of ribeye slices in hot broth until medium-rare, 10 to 20 seconds per batch.

Step 3

Bring a large pot of water to a boil. Add noodles; cook at a boil until tender, 3 to 5 minutes. Drain.

Step 4

Place tortillas on a microwave-safe plate. Heat in the microwave until warm, 20 to 25 seconds.

Step 5

Divide onion and jalapeno mixture, ribeye slices, noodles, chili-garlic sauce, bean sprouts, hoisin sauce, Thai basil, and cilantro among warmed tortillas. Spoon a small amount of broth on top. Fold opposing edges of tortillas over filling and roll up into burritos. Serve with lime slices.

Nutrition Facts

Per Serving: 248 calories; protein 15.1g; carbohydrates 68.7g; fat 12g; cholesterol 20.4mg; sodium 1939.6mg.

## Basic Vegetarian Pho

I adapted this Asian pho dish from a traditional Hmong recipe for my vegetarian fiance. The broth is very basic and then each person seasons and garnishes it according to their individual tastes. There is no right way to season and garnish this dish. Be creative and feel free to add your own twist. For flavoring, use red pepper paste, soy sauce, teriyaki sauce, and sesame oil.

Prep: 20 mins

Cook: 30 mins

Additional: 10 mins

Total: 1 hr

Servings: 8

Yield: 8 servings

Ingredients

Broth:

3 (32 fluid ounce) containers vegetable broth

6 stalks lemon grass, cut into 1-inch pieces

2 tablespoons vegetable bouillon (such as Better Than Bouillon®)

5 whole star anise pods

Noodles and Garnish:

1 (16 ounce) package dried thin rice noodles

1 (8 ounce) package bean sprouts

1 (8 ounce) package sliced fresh mushrooms

2 limes, sliced, or as desired

1 bunch fresh cilantro

1 (.75 ounce) package fresh basil

1 bunch green onions, sliced

Flavoring:

¼ cup teriyaki sauce, or to taste

¼ cup soy sauce, or to taste

¼ cup chile paste, or to taste

¼ cup sesame oil, or to taste

Directions

Step 1

Combine vegetable broth, lemon grass, vegetable bouillon, and star anise pods in a saucepan and bring to a boil. Reduce heat and let simmer until flavors are combined, 30 to 45 minutes. Remove lemon grass and star anise with a slotted spoon and discard.

Step 2

Place rice noodles in a bowl and cover with hot water to soften, about 10 minutes. Drain and cut into shorter pieces with kitchen shears; divide noodles equally between soup bowls. Fill bowls with hot broth to cover noodles.

Step 3

Place bean sprouts, mushrooms, limes, cilantro, basil, and green onions into separate bowls. Place teriyaki sauce, soy sauce, chile paste, and sesame oil in separate bowls. Serve soup alongside garnishes and flavorings.

Nutrition Facts

Per Serving: 287 calories; protein 7.5g; carbohydrates 71.3g; fat 9.3g; sodium 1669.2mg.

## Pho Ga Soup

Vietnamese chicken noodle soup. After ordering this soup at a local Vietnamese restaurant, I decided to try to make it at home. This is a very flexible recipe. Feel free to substitute some of your favorite vegetables or try different noodles. Enjoy!

Prep: 15 mins

Cook: 15 mins

Total: 30 mins

Servings: 6

Yield: 6 servings

Ingredients

1 tablespoon vegetable oil

1 small yellow onion, chopped

1 (8 ounce) package baby bella mushrooms, chopped

4 cloves garlic, minced

8 cups water

1 (6.75 ounce) package rice stick noodles (such as Maifun®)

8 teaspoons chicken bouillon

2 cooked chicken breasts, shredded

4 green onions, chopped

⅓ cup chopped fresh cilantro

2 cups bean sprouts

1 lime, sliced into wedges

1 dash Sriracha hot sauce, or more to taste

Directions

Step 1

Heat vegetable oil in a large saucepan over medium-high heat; saute onion, mushrooms, and garlic until tender, 5 to 10 minutes. Add water, rice noodles, and chicken bouillon to onion mixture; bring to a boil. Reduce heat to low.

Step 2

Mix shredded chicken, green onions, and cilantro into soup; simmer for 5 minutes more. Transfer soup to serving bowls and top with bean sprouts, a squeeze of lime juice, and Sriracha hot sauce.

Nutrition Facts

Per Serving: 231 calories; protein 13.5g; carbohydrates 32g; fat 5.4g; cholesterol 27.5mg; sodium 148.9mg.

Very healthy soup! I came up with the idea myself and, once I tried it, I knew that I had a winner here. It is somewhat spicy and is very, very good for if you have a cold, would like to warm up in the winter, or to clear your nose.

Prep: 15 mins

Cook: 1 hr 48 mins

Total: 2 hrs 3 mins

Servings: 8

Yield: 8 servings

Ingredients

2 teaspoons sesame oil, divided

1 (4 inch) piece fresh ginger, peeled and chopped, or to taste

3 quarts chicken broth

1 large red onion, diced

2 cups sliced carrots

1 tablespoon curry powder

1 tablespoon ground ginger

1 tablespoon cayenne pepper

salt and ground black pepper to taste

1 jalapeno pepper, finely chopped

6 limes, juiced, divided

1 (9 ounce) package udon noodles

4 skinless, boneless chicken breast halves, cubed

1 leek, cut into matchstick-size pieces

1 green onion, finely chopped

Directions

Step 1

Heat 1 teaspoon sesame oil in a large pot over low heat; cook and stir ginger in the hot oil for 10 minutes. Pour chicken broth over ginger, cover pot, and simmer for 30 minutes.

Step 2

Stir onion and carrots into broth and simmer until carrots are tender, about 10 minutes. Gradually add curry powder, ground ginger, cayenne pepper, salt, and black pepper to broth; stir in jalapeno pepper and half the lime juice. Simmer broth over low heat, stirring about every 15 minutes, until flavors have blended, about 1 hour.

Step 3

Fill a large pot with lightly salted water and bring to a rolling boil. Drop udon in a few noodles at a time and return to a boil. Cook uncovered, stirring occasionally, until the pasta has cooked through, but is still firm to the bite, 10 to 12 minutes; drain.

Step 4

Heat 1 teaspoon sesame oil in a skillet over medium heat; cook and stir chicken in the hot oil until no longer pink in the center, about 10 minutes. Transfer chicken to broth and stir leek and green onion into broth; simmer for 5 to 10 more minutes. Remove pot from heat.

Step 5

Portion udon noodles into each serving bowl; ladle broth over noodles. Add remaining lime juice to each serving.

Nutrition Facts

Per Serving: 225 calories; protein 15.8g; carbohydrates 30.6g; fat 4g; cholesterol 36.8mg; sodium 1701.9mg.

## Vegetarian Pho (Vietnamese Noodle Soup)

A vegetarian version of this tasty Vietnamese noodle soup.

Prep: 30 mins

Cook: 1 hr 4 mins

Total: 1 hr 34 mins

Servings: 6

Yield: 6 bowls

Ingredients

Broth:

10 cups vegetable stock

1 onion, peeled and halved

¼ cup soy sauce

8 cloves garlic, coarsely chopped

2 (3 inch) cinnamon sticks

2 teaspoons ground ginger

2 pods star anise

2 bay leaves

Soup:

1 (16 ounce) package thin rice noodles (such as Thai Kitchen®)

2 tablespoons vegetable oil, or as needed

2 (14 ounce) packages firm tofu, drained and cut into 1/4-inch slices

8 ounces enoki mushrooms

4 scallions, thinly sliced

½ cup coarsely chopped cilantro

1 lime, cut into wedges

2 jalapeno peppers, sliced into rings

¼ cup mung bean sprouts

¼ cup Thai basil leaves, torn into bite-size pieces

Directions

Step 1

Place vegetable stock, onion, soy sauce, garlic, cinnamon sticks, ground ginger, star anise, and bay leaves in a large pot; bring to a boil. Reduce heat, cover, and simmer until flavors combine, 30 to 45 minutes. Remove solids with a slotted spoon and keep broth hot.

Step 2

Place noodles in a large bowl and cover with boiling water. Set aside until noodles are softened, 8 to 10 minutes. Drain and rinse thoroughly. Divide noodles among 6 serving bowls.

Step 3

Heat oil in a large skillet over medium-high heat until shimmering. Add tofu in a single layer and fry, in batches, until golden brown, about 6 minutes per side.

Step 4

Simmer fried tofu and mushrooms in broth until heated through, about 5 minutes. Transfer to serving bowls. Top with scallions and cilantro. Ladle in hot broth.

Step 5

Serve lime wedges, jalapeno peppers, bean sprouts, and basil alongside for garnishing each bowl.

Nutrition Facts

Per Serving: 283 calories; protein 16.6g; carbohydrates 77.7g; fat 12.6g; sodium 1208.8mg.

## CONCLUSION

Pho is a Vietnamese soup made with broth, rice noodles, herbs, and meat or tofu. Due to its nutritious ingredients and high protein content, it may offer several benefits, including reduced inflammation and improved joint health. Still, it can be high in sodium and calories, so portion size is important. Overall, pho can be a nutritious addition to a well-balanced diet.